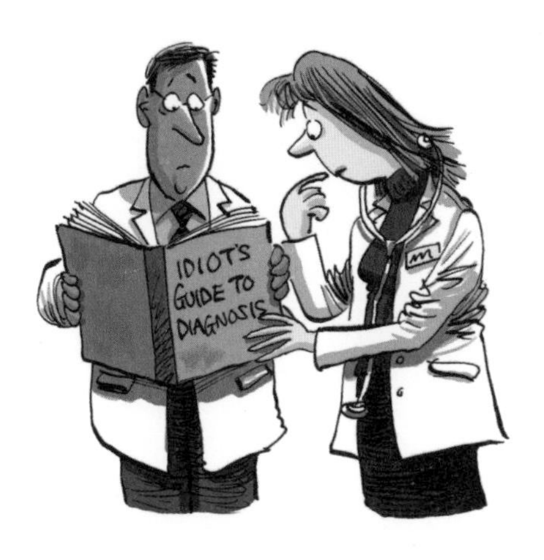

How to Survive Being a
DOCTOR

CLIVE WHICHELOW *and* MIKE HASKINS

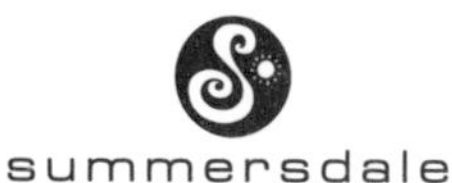
summersdale

HOW TO SURVIVE BEING A DOCTOR

Illustrations by Ian Baker

Summersdale Publishers Ltd
46 West Street
Chichester
West Sussex
PO19 1RP
UK

www.summersdale.com

Printed and bound in China

ISBN: 978-1-78685-252-6

To.................................

From.............................

Introduction

Open your mouth and say 'ahhh' – or, if you're a doctor, open your mouth and say 'aaarrrgghhh'!

Yes, as a doctor you have to deal with soppy patients, stroppy patients, hypochondriacs, time-wasters, chatterers, unruly children, unruly pensioners, people who have researched their condition on the internet and tell you that you don't know what you're talking about, people who are determined to get their money's worth out of the NHS (whether they're ill or not) and people who are inconveniently ill just when you are about to go home.

Yes, all human life is there, and some inhuman life too. But wouldn't it be boring otherwise? Imagine if no one ever got ill.

You'd be sitting around in your ward or surgery staring at the walls and dishing out flu jabs and leaflets about 'five a day' till kingdom come. The only patients you'd ever see would be other doctors suffering the screaming abdabs from having nothing to do all day.

Frustration, tension and botheration come with the territory, but along with them come laughs, human interest and drama. Like a good night on the telly used to have.

You will have the fun of refusing a sick note to someone who tells you they have laryngitis – when you reply that he can't have, because he just told you – or to someone who strides into the surgery to tell you an accident has left them unable to walk.

It will be fabulous. All you need to do is learn the survival techniques.

TYPES OF DOCTOR YOU COULD BE

Confident and welcoming, so your patients feel you are pleased to see them

• • • • • • • • • • •

Easy-going and cheerful, so your patients leave feeling happier than when they came in

ARROGANT AND SELF-SATISFIED, SO YOUR PATIENTS SUSPECT YOUR PRIMARY INTEREST IS TO FIND THEY HAVE CONTRACTED A PREVIOUSLY UNKNOWN DISEASE WHICH YOU CAN THEN HAVE NAMED AFTER YOURSELF

Negative and paranoid,
so that you believe
even a runny nose
must be the first sign
of the Black Death

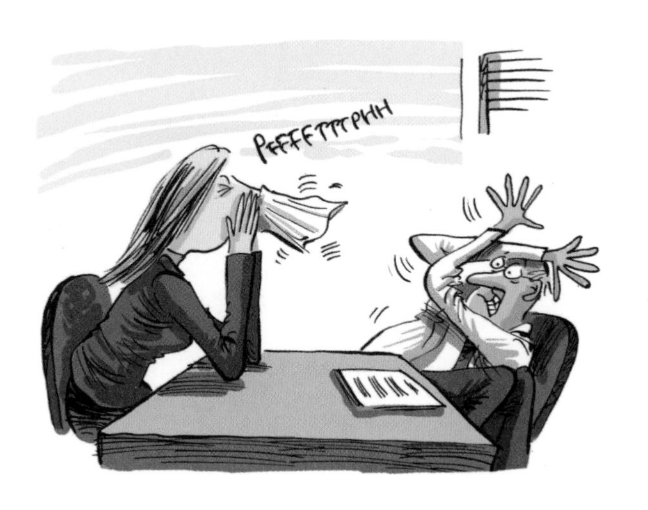
PFFFFTTTPHH

WAYS TO CONVINCE PATIENTS THAT YOU KNOW WHAT YOU'RE DOING

Whatever condition they come in with, say you've had exactly the same

• • • • • • • • • •

Perfect a way of looking things up on the computer without them noticing

• • • • • • • • • •

Nod knowledgeably while they are describing their symptoms, even though inwardly you're completely baffled

LOOK IMPRESSED BY WHATEVER'S WRONG WITH THEM AS THOUGH GETTING ILL WAS A GREAT ACHIEVEMENT ON THEIR PART

GIVEAWAYS THAT WILL CONVINCE PATIENTS YOU DON'T KNOW WHAT YOU'RE DOING

You look horrified by whatever's wrong with them and run out of the room shrieking in terror

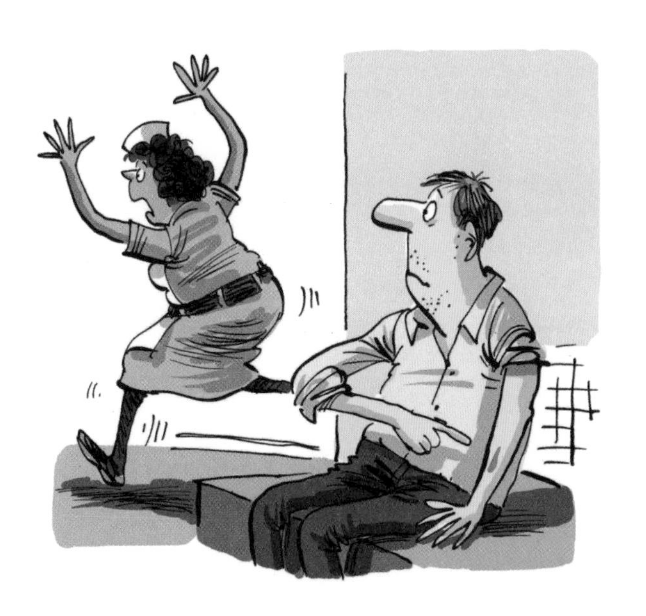

You are clearly suffering from the same condition that they have

• • • • • • • • • •

You ask them to spell out, letter by letter, the illness that they have so you can look it up

• • • • • • • • • •

You lose interest and nod off while they are describing their symptoms

GOOD ROLE MODELS FOR DOCTORS

Doctor Quinn, Medicine Woman – able to make a diagnosis even when under attack from rattlesnakes and bears

• • • • • • • • • • •

Doctor Dana Scully – never forgetting that there must be some kind of logical explanation for even the most bizarre symptoms

• • • • • • • • • • •

Doctor McCoy – a good all-rounder who doesn't need to drive to appointments – he can just beam down to the patient's bedside instead

Doctor Who – able to solve even the most complex problems with a single, highly sophisticated instrument

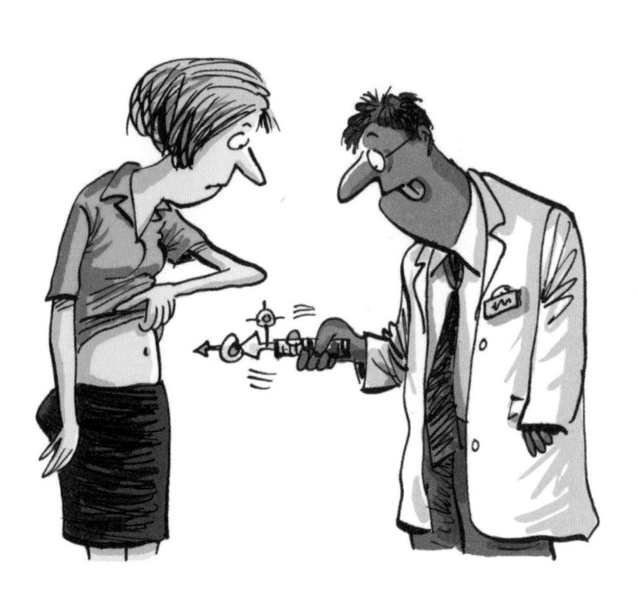

FANTASY AND REALITY OF HOW YOU WILL BE REGARDED AS A DOCTOR

FANTASY	REALITY
A trusted person who is almost a member of the family	'Not the same doctor I saw last time'
A medical expert that has the answer to every known condition	A know-nothing plonker that won't dish out sick notes on demand
A person whose advice should be listened to carefully and taken seriously	A person whose advice is secondary to the presenters on breakfast television
Someone who will fully respect patient confidentiality	Someone who might suddenly whip out a camera and start filming an episode of *Embarrassing Bodies*

A SELECTION OF DOCTORS' ACRONYMS FOR PATIENTS

BIFFA	Browsed Internet, Found Fatal Ailment
VINI	Vivid Imagination, Not Ill
PITA BREAD	Pain In The A*** – Bad Reaction to Every Available Drug
OCTWATT	Only Comes To While Away The Time
BIMMBBO	Belief In Miracles Might Be Best Option
WOMBAT	Waste Of Medication, Believes in Alternative Therapies
GOFDAROP	Good Only For Dismantling And Recycling Of Parts

LOLINOTROW: LITTLE OLD LADY IN NEED OF TOTAL REPLACEMENT OF WATERWORKS

BAD ROLE MODELS FOR DOCTORS

Doctor Dolittle – would probably prefer working with animals

• • • • • • • • • • •

Doctor Zira from *Planet of the Apes* – has a worrying fondness for lobotomies

• • • • • • • • • • •

Doctor Hannibal Lecter – that mask he wears may not be able to stop the spread of germs

Doctor Frankenstein – dangerous and possibly insane, although willing to recycle discarded parts from previous patients

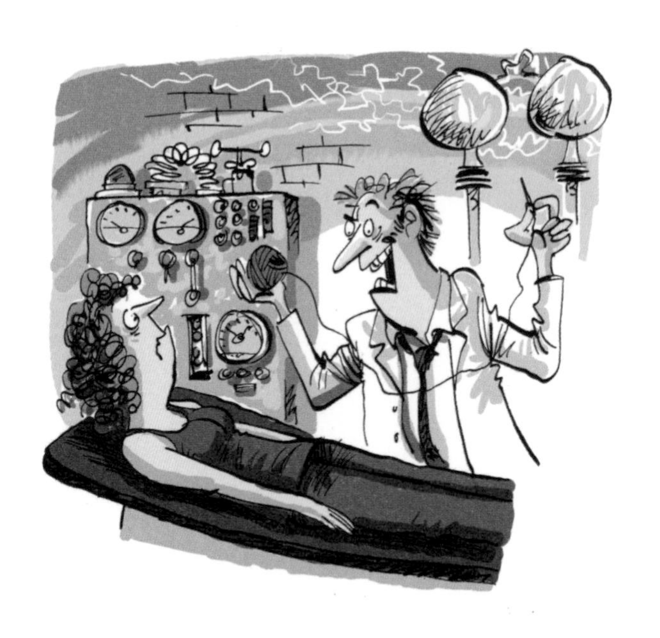

BREAKDOWN OF HOW TIME IS SPENT DURING THE DOCTOR'S DAY

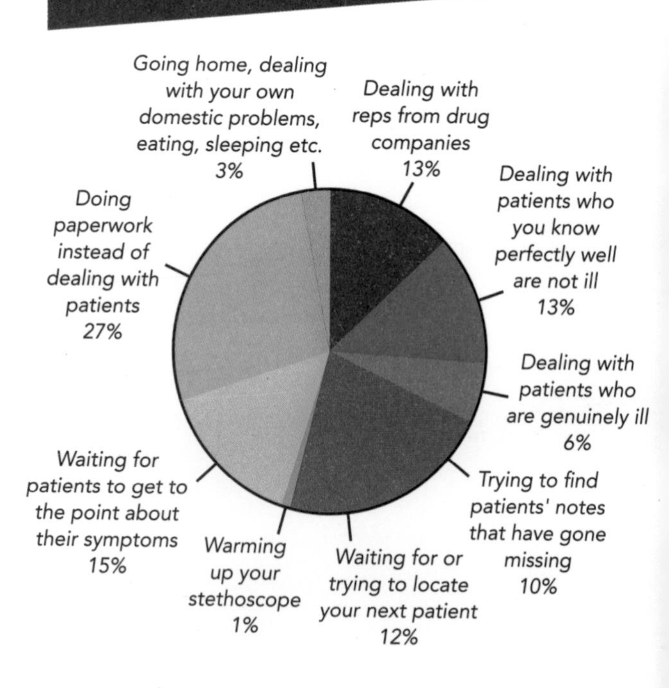

THINGS YOU SHOULD AND SHOULDN'T SAY TO PATIENTS

SHOULD SAY	SHOULDN'T SAY
There's really nothing to worry about	Is your life insurance up to date?
What seems to be the trouble?	Oh no, not you again!
Where exactly does it hurt?	Do you have anywhere at all where it doesn't hurt?
I'm going to try you on some new medication	If you survive swallowing this bottle of tablets I'll get a nice bonus from the manufacturer

IMPORTANT THINGS YOU MAY FIND YOURSELF WORRYING ABOUT

That you simply don't have enough time to spend with each patient

• • • • • • • • • • •

That you have life-and-death decisions to make on a daily basis

• • • • • • • • • • •

How to adopt the appropriate tone when giving a patient their test results

WHETHER YOU
HAVE THE LATEST,
MOST APPROPRIATE
DIAGNOSTIC TOOLS
AVAILABLE

LESS IMPORTANT THINGS YOU WILL FIND YOURSELF WORRYING ABOUT

That you simply don't have enough time in which to play rounds of golf

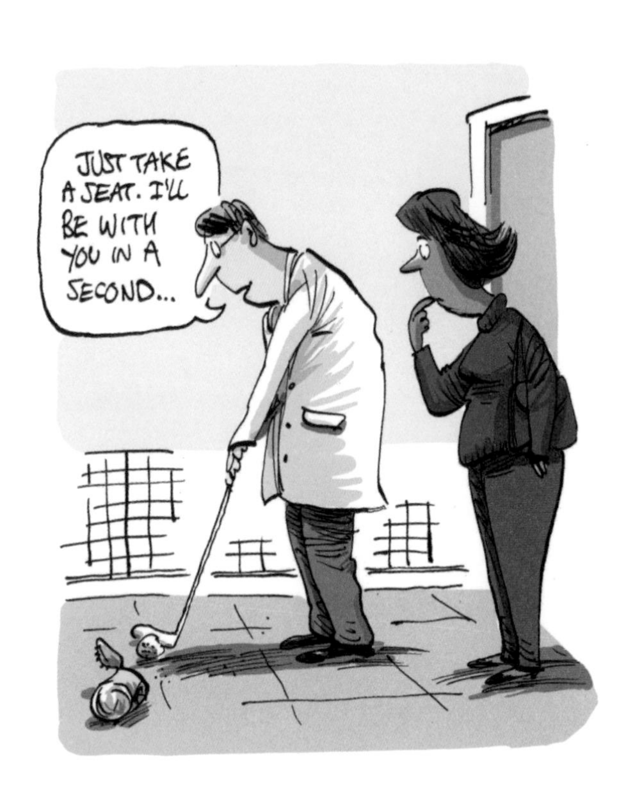
JUST TAKE A SEAT. I'LL BE WITH YOU IN A SECOND...

Whether your decision to have full-fat milk in your tea is a bad example to patients

• • • • • • • • • • •

How to adopt the right pose to be found in when the next patient enters your consulting room

• • • • • • • • • • •

Whether to wear your stethoscope trailing over one shoulder or casually hanging out of your pocket

THINGS DOCTORS END UP WITH IN THEIR HOMES

DVDs of fictional television doctors that present the state-of-the-art working conditions, perfect patients and glamorous colleagues they are sadly lacking

• • • • • • • • • • •

A patient's urine sample which is the exact colour wanted for the spare room

• • • • • • • • • • •

Freebies from drug companies which will serve as Christmas presents for their least-favourite relatives

Extraordinary growths that they have personally removed from patients and which they now gleefully exhibit to any visitors

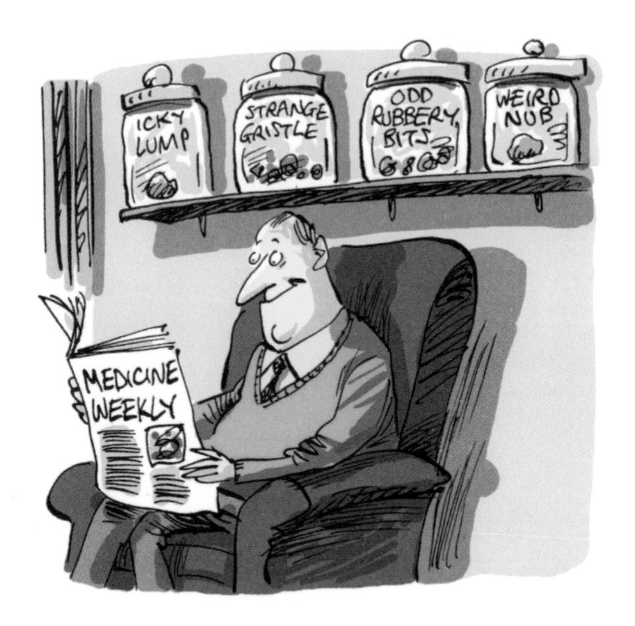
ICKY LUMP
STRANGE GRISTLE
ODD RUBBERY BITS
WEIRD NUB
MEDICINE WEEKLY

DOs AND DON'Ts DURING PATIENT CONSULTATIONS

Do try to avoid making your patient feel self-conscious if they have to undress for an examination

Don't be tempted to whip off your own kit as well, just to keep them company

• • • • • • • • • • •

Do prescribe medication carefully and as appropriate

Don't write the patient a blank prescription and tell them to fill their boots just to get rid of them

DO SEEK A SECOND OPINION IF YOU FEEL THIS IS APPROPRIATE

DON'T SIT IN FRONT OF THE PATIENT THUMBING THROUGH THE *READER'S DIGEST MEDICAL ENCYCLOPAEDIA* TRYING TO WORK OUT WHAT'S WRONG WITH THEM

Do remember to remain calm and collected when a patient shows you an unusual rash or swelling

Don't pull out your phone to take a photo while exclaiming: 'Blimey! This'll really gross my mates out when I put it up on Facebook.'

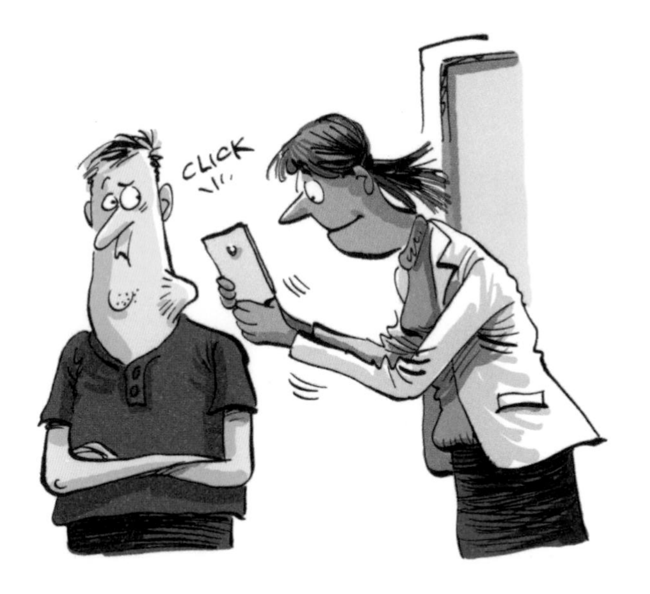
CLICK

INADVISABLE SHORTCUTS

Writing out a prescription for antibiotics before the patient has even had a chance to explain their symptoms

• • • • • • • • • • •

Getting the patients in two at a time to save valuable minutes

• • • • • • • • • • •

Asking your patients to draw a picture of themselves naked rather than having to endure the sight of them stripping off for examination

SPRAYING YOUR PATIENTS WITH DDT AND PUTTING THEM THROUGH A SHEEP DIP BEFORE YOU'LL TOUCH THEM

REALISTIC AND UNREALISTIC GOALS

REALISTIC	UNREALISTIC
To be able to cure some of your patients some of the time	For your surgery or clinic to be comparable to Lourdes as a place of healing and pilgrimage
To be thanked occasionally by grateful patients	To be made a beneficiary in the wills of all your patients – particularly the ones who are very elderly and extremely well off
You will play some small part in making your local community fitter and healthier	You will single-handedly transform your local community into a new race of super beings
You will make a contribution to medical science that will be remembered in years to come	For future generations, your name will be synonymous with the term 'doctor'

EMOTIONAL RESPONSES YOU SHOULD PRACTISE

'Genuine' sympathy for when a patient tells you exactly how long they've been sitting in the waiting room

• • • • • • • • • • •

Your poker face for when being presented with a self-inflicted injury that is utterly hilarious

• • • • • • • • • • •

Stoicism for when greeting the hypochondriac who books an appointment every few days

X-Factor-style bigged-up delight for when a patient's test results come back negative

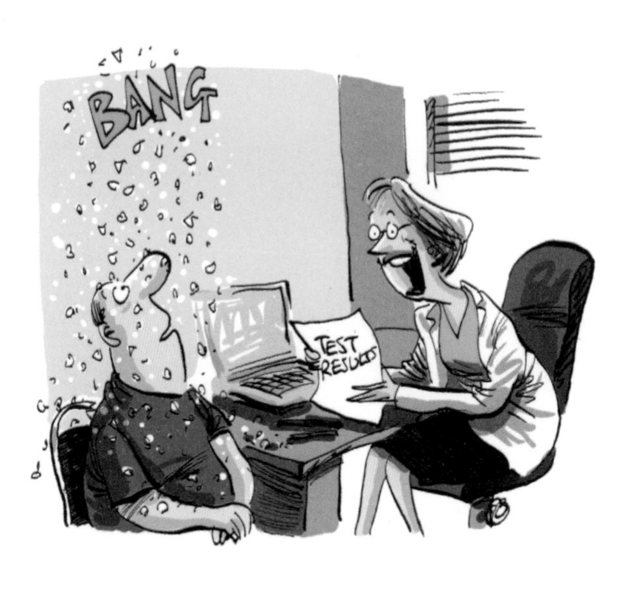
BANG
TEST

HABITS
YOU SHOULD AVOID

Breaking into uncontrollable laughter when someone describes their symptoms

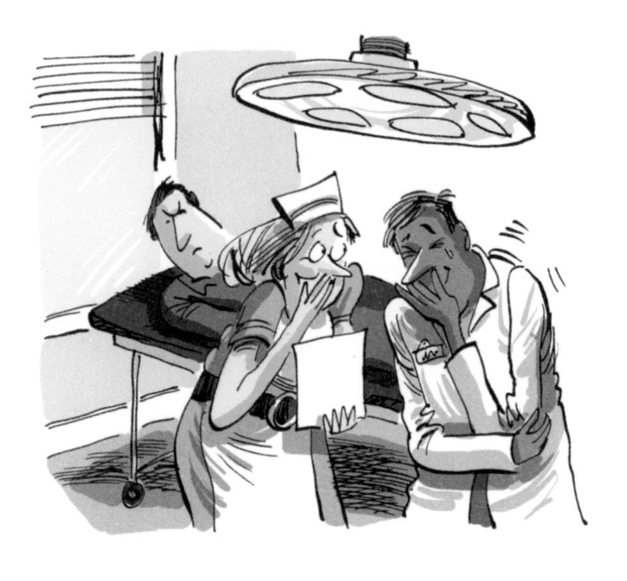

Saying 'this won't hurt a bit' when
you know damn well that it will

• • • • • • • • • • •

Wiping a tongue depressor on your
backside before using it on a patient

• • • • • • • • • • •

Putting your stethoscope in the
fridge before seeing a patient you
don't particularly care for

GOOD AND BAD INTERIOR DECOR FOR THE DOCTOR'S SURGERY

GOOD	BAD
Gentle pastel shades that make the patient feel relaxed	Luminous paint that can be seen from the next street
Some tasteful watercolours on the walls	A Damien Hirst installation of a rotting animal
Some nice pot plants	Some nice 'pot' plants for patients to use as an alternative form of pain relief
A clock that shows the length of time your next patient has left to wait for their appointment	A clock that shows the amount of time your next patient has left on this Earth

CHANGES
THAT WILL OCCUR IN YOUR APPEARANCE

You will have a permanently furrowed brow from having to look concerned as patients reel off their various complaints and conditions

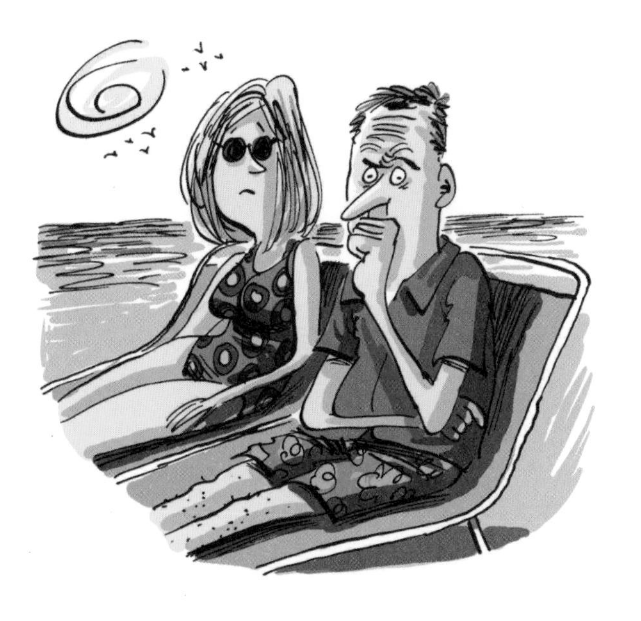

You will have a permanent squint from
having one eye on the patient and the
other simultaneously on the computer

• • • • • • • • • • •

You will put your neck out from making
too big a show of looking away while
a patient adjusts their clothing

• • • • • • • • • • •

Because of lack of sleep, you will develop
bags under your eyes big enough
to hold your medical equipment

READY RESPONSES FOR THINGS YOUR PATIENTS WILL SAY

'I'm not a hypochondriac' – 'Perhaps you just think that you aren't!'

• • • • • • • • • •

'Have I got anything serious, Doctor?' – 'That depends: how good is your sense of humour?'

• • • • • • • • • •

'So I don't need to make another appointment. That's good news then!' – 'You don't – but I'm afraid it isn't!'

• • • • • • • • • •

'This is a bit embarrassing, doctor' – 'It won't be embarrassing for me!'

THE DOCTOR'S WARDROBE – A GUIDE TO WHAT TO WEAR AND WHAT NOT TO WEAR

WEAR	DON'T WEAR
Something smart that gives a patient confidence in you as a professional	Something lairy that gives the patient a headache with all the clashing colours
A friendly smile that helps patients think you are sympathetic	A look of disbelief that makes patients think they have a condition which will baffle the entire medical profession
Something clean and clinical	An all-over environmental protection suit
Loose casual clothes to put your patients at ease when you examine them	Clothes that are so loose your patients can see enough to examine you

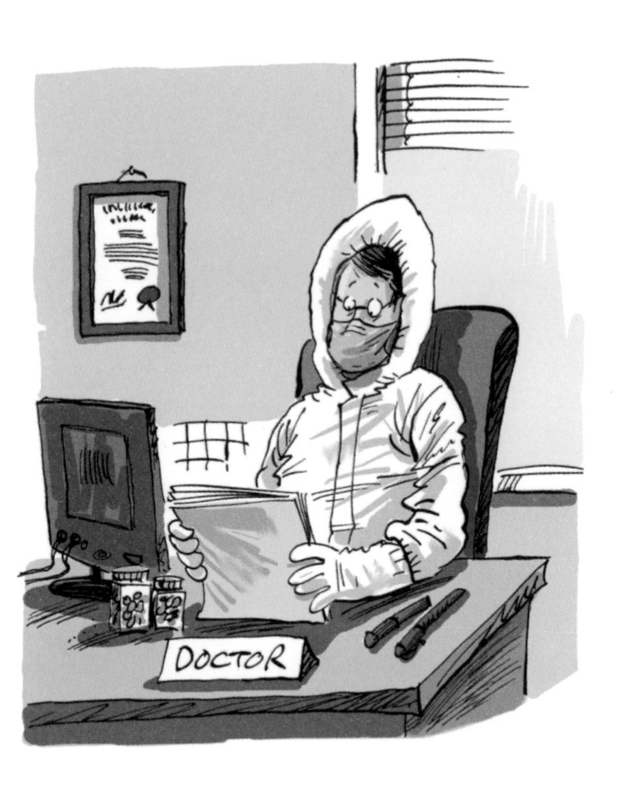
DOCTOR

WAYS IN WHICH YOUR PATIENTS MAY ENDANGER YOUR HEALTH

They will drive you to drinking, smoking, fast food and all the other things you warn them against

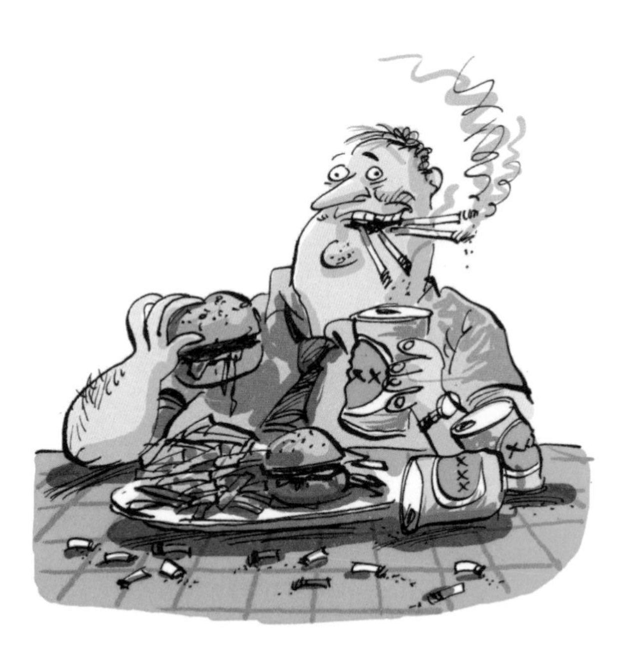

You will become convinced that you have half the health issues that you are hearing from them every day of the week

• • • • • • • • • • •

You get concussed when the heavy medical book you are reaching for falls off the shelf straight onto your head

• • • • • • • • • • •

You accidentally close your consulting-room door on your own fingers while attempting to gently chivvy them out

ADVANTAGES AND DISADVANTAGES OF BEING A DOCTOR

ADVANTAGE	DISADVANTAGE
You earn a good salary	You never have any time to spend it
You have the power of life and death in your hands	You have the power of life and death in your hands
You get to meet lots of different, interesting people	Every single one of them is ill
You can make a real difference to people's lives	If you're not careful, it might not be in a good way

THOUGHTS
THAT WILL CAUSE YOU UNNECESSARY STRESS

When is the polite moment to don a face mask when you find yourself in the presence of a particularly contagious patient?

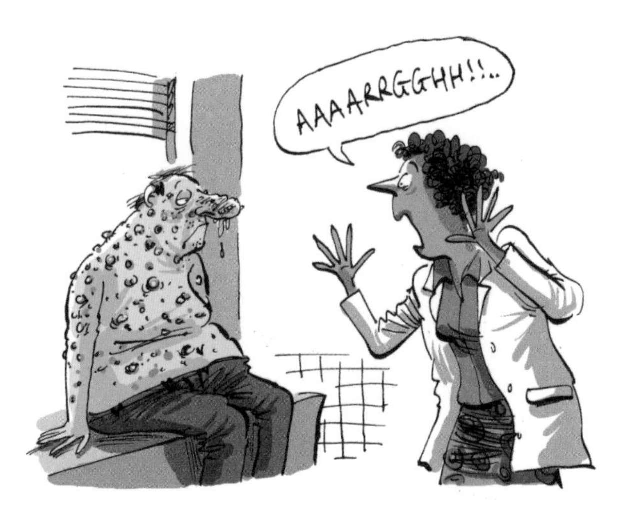
AAAARRGGHH!!..

When you're ill, you can only go
to someone like yourself!

• • • • • • • • • •

Why are all the bosses of drug
companies richer than you are?

• • • • • • • • • •

Trying to remember those two or three
things you never bothered revising
for your finals at medical school

ACTIVITIES YOU SHOULDN'T ENGAGE IN WHEN WITH A PATIENT

Checking how your online auction bids are doing

• • • • • • • • • • •

Chuckling over a funny clip someone has sent you on Facebook

• • • • • • • • • • •

Using your consulting room sink to go to the lavatory

Clipping your toenails

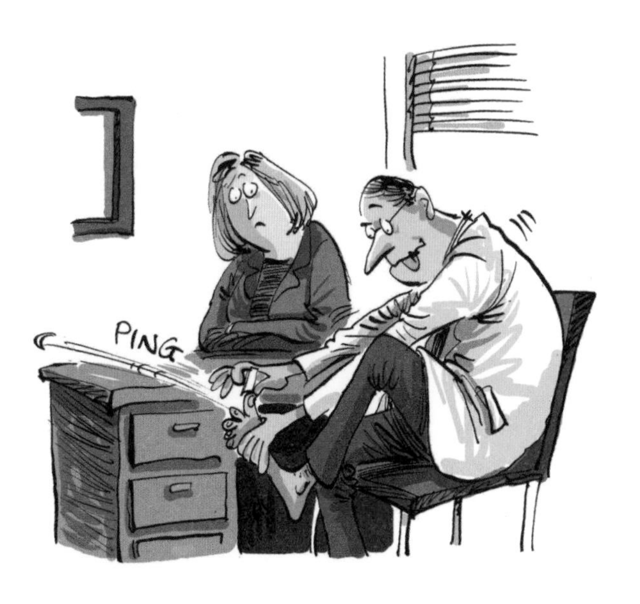
PING

SELF-HELP BOOKS FOR DOCTORS

How to Translate Hypochondriac Fantasies into Plain English

• • • • • • • • • •

How to Stay Patient With Your Patients

• • • • • • • • • •

A Beginner's Guide to Deciphering Your Own Handwriting

• • • • • • • • • •

The British Pharmacopoeia Supplement on the Best Placebos to Get Rid of Persistent Patients for a Day or Two

BREAKDOWN OF A DOCTOR'S EXPENDITURE

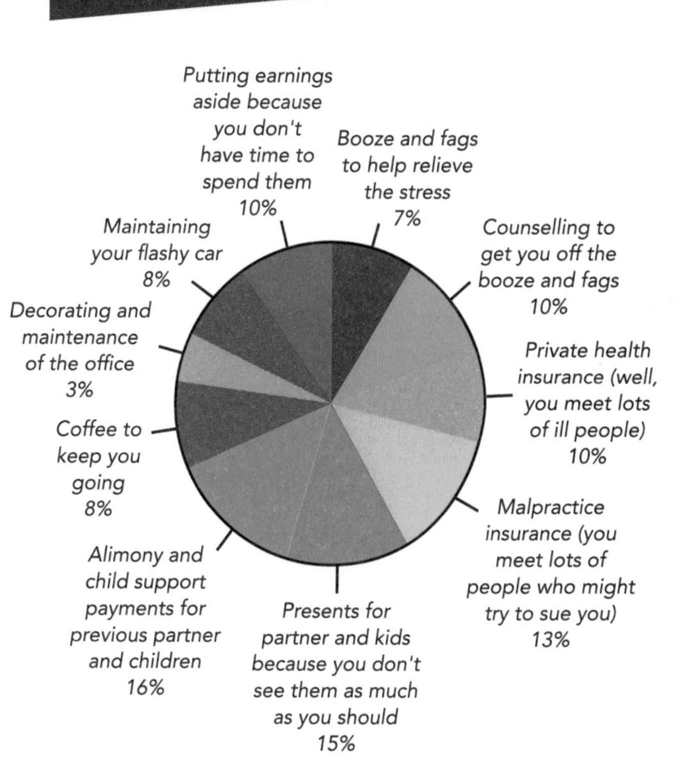

PROBLEMS
ARISING FROM MISREADING PATIENTS' NOTES

Treating a patient who you thought was 'profoundly dead' rather than 'profoundly deaf'

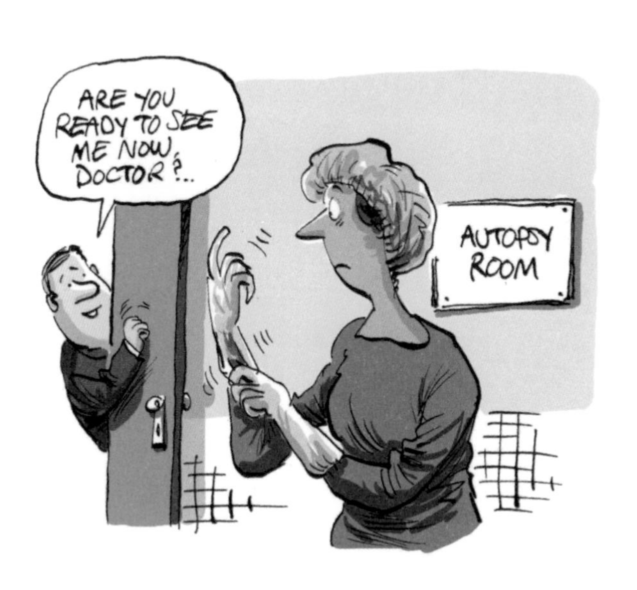
ARE YOU READY TO SEE ME NOW, DOCTOR?..
AUTOPSY ROOM

Trying to work out why the
tattooed bricklayer in front of you
wants breast enhancements

• • • • • • • • • • •

Misreading 'highly contagious'
as 'hardly contagious'

• • • • • • • • • • •

Preparing to perform an autopsy on
a patient who actually came in for an
'automatic prescription renewal'

INADVISABLE WAYS TO USE BEING A DOCTOR TO YOUR ADVANTAGE

Wearing a white coat at all times in the hope of shop discounts

• • • • • • • • • • •

Selling off sick notes from work to the highest bidder on eBay

• • • • • • • • • • •

Telling your most irritating patient that they have a potentially fatal allergy which could be triggered by going too near a doctor

Hailing ambulances instead of taxis for lifts home from the pub

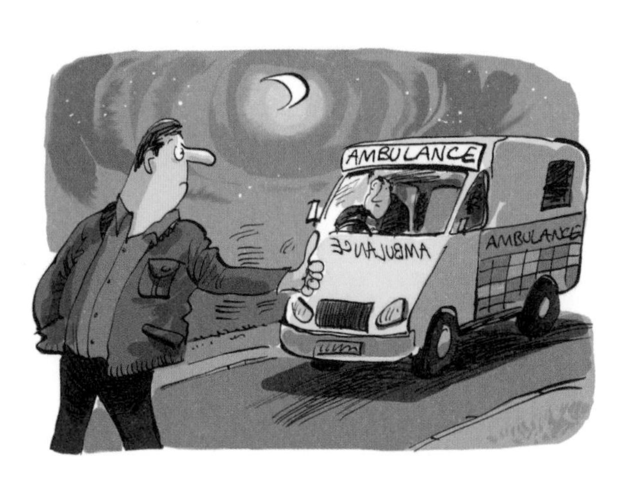
AMBULANCE
AMBULANCE

THINGS YOU FIND YOURSELF SAYING NOW

'And what seems to be the matter?' – even if it's just the window-cleaner calling

• • • • • • • • • • •

'How many units of alcohol do you drink a week?' – quite annoying for the other drinkers in the pub

• • • • • • • • • • •

'Would you like a sticker that says "I was very brave at the doctors today"' – okay when treating small children; not okay after a visit from friends or family

‘OKAY, POP YOUR TOP
OFF FOR ME
AND LET’S HAVE A
LITTLE LOOK-SEE!’
– ESPECIALLY
INAPPROPRIATE
WHEN IN BED WITH
YOUR PARTNER

HOW PEOPLE WILL KNOW YOU'RE A DOCTOR

You have magazine subscriptions to an extensive and odd mixture of titles, including Reader's Digest, Men's Health, Golf Monthly, Woman's Realm, The People's Friend, The World of Interiors and The Beano

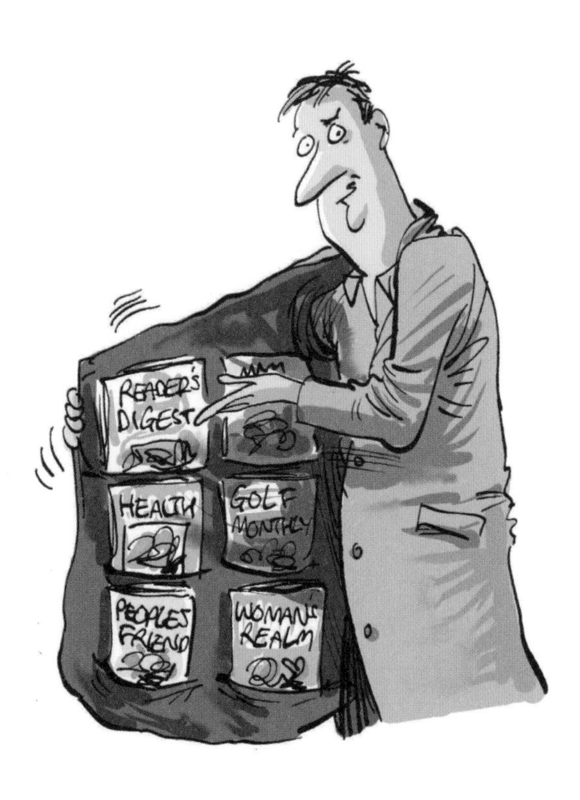
READER'S DIGEST
HEALTH
GOLF MONTHLY
PEOPLES FRIEND
WOMAN'S REALM

Your eyes glaze over when anyone mentions their health problems

• • • • • • • • • •

You're the only person they know who never complains about GP waiting times

• • • • • • • • • •

Whenever you get bored with someone, you try writing a prescription to get them to go away

THINGS YOU REALLY SHOULDN'T SAY NOW

'How are you?' – because if people know you're a doctor they will tell you (at great length)

• • • • • • • • • • •

'Good health!' – if a doctor says this before knocking back a double whisky, onlookers may take it as official medical advice

• • • • • • • • • • •

'Looking forward to Christmas?' – people will take this to mean that you've spotted some reason they are unlikely to make it to then

PROFILE
OF AN IDEAL PATIENT

Someone who only comes to see you once a year – and that's to give you a bottle of something nice for Christmas

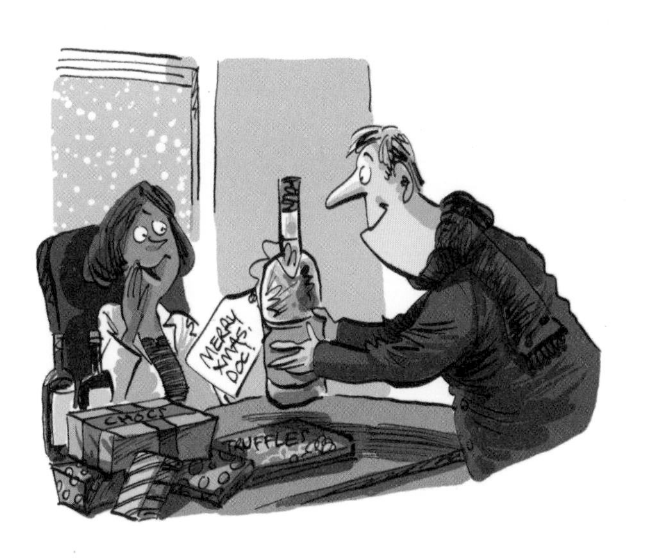
MERRY XMAS DOC!
CHOCS
TRUFFLES

Someone with such a weak bladder they are unable to hang around for very long

• • • • • • • • • •

Someone with no conversational skills and a massively obvious (but easily treatable) problem

• • • • • • • • • •

Someone who has waited so long to see you that they have already got better

THINGS ONLY A DOCTOR WOULD FIND EXCITING

The latest issue of *The Lancet*

• • • • • • • • • • •

Finding their own name mentioned in the latest issue of *The Lancet*

• • • • • • • • • • •

A particularly large and misshapen lump in a highly unexpected place

• • • • • • • • • • •

The latest developments in artificial-hip-replacement technology

PROFILE
OF THE PATIENT FROM HELL

Someone who comes out with an apparently never-ending series of problems and symptoms, like a magician producing flags of all nations from his sleeve

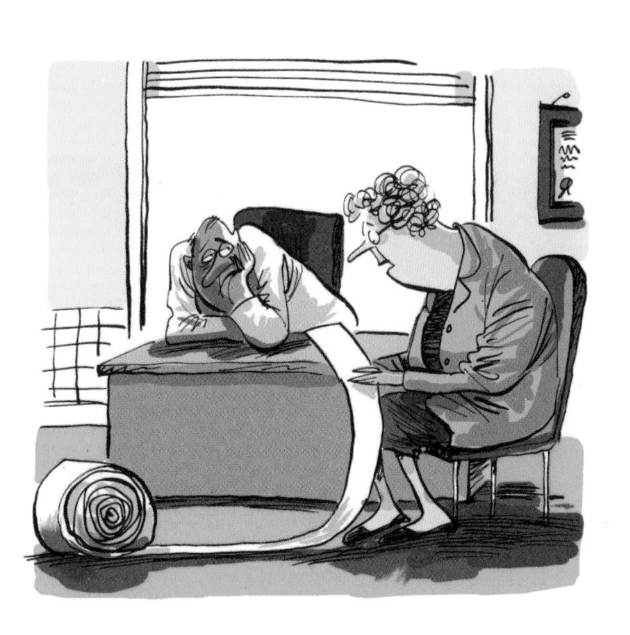

Someone who comes to see you every other week – mainly to complain about the treatment they got last time

• • • • • • • • • • •

Someone whose main medical complaint seems to be an allergy to soap and water

• • • • • • • • • • •

Someone who seems reluctant to find their way back out of your consulting room

THINGS ONLY A DOCTOR WOULD DREAD

A cure for the common cold
– mass redundancies!

• • • • • • • • • • •

The reintroduction of home visits

• • • • • • • • • • •

A patient who brings one or more friends along to sit in during their appointment

Patients who present you with a wad of print-outs from the internet detailing their condition together with a shopping list of medication and procedures

GOOD WAYS FOR A DOCTOR TO RELAX

A glass of wine and a nice meal

• • • • • • • • • •

A gentle walk in the countryside

• • • • • • • • • •

A nice long drive far away from work

Reading the magazines
left in the waiting room

BAD WAYS FOR A DOCTOR TO RELAX

A bottle of Scotch and a takeaway

• • • • • • • • • • •

A disturbed walk in their sleep

• • • • • • • • • • •

Racing anxiously all the way back to work because they have just been notified of an emergency that they need to deal with

Performing forensic analysis of the germs left all over the magazines in the waiting room

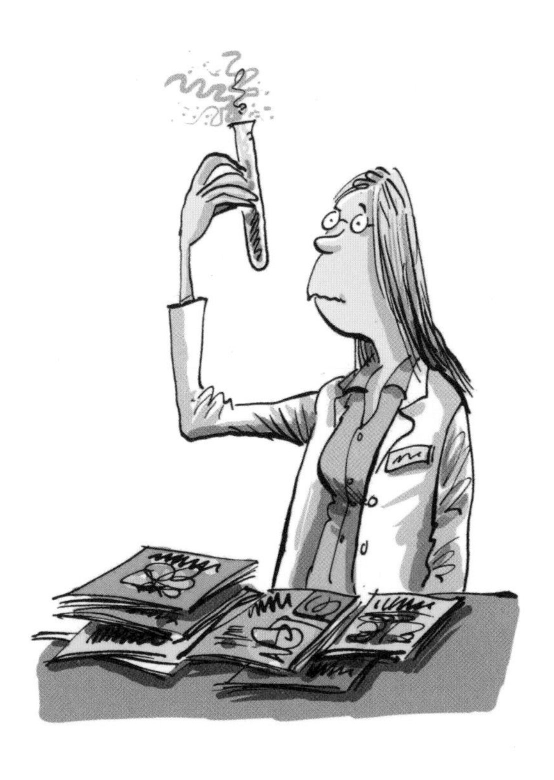

THINGS YOU MIGHT HAVE IN YOUR LITTLE BLACK BAG

A stethoscope (don't forget to warm it up)

• • • • • • • • • • •

A thermometer (don't mix up oral and rectal)

• • • • • • • • • • •

A specimen bottle (preferably clean)

• • • • • • • • • • •

A wad of prescription forms (don't fill them out ready like a book of blank cheques)

THINGS YOU SHOULDN'T HAVE IN YOUR LITTLE BLACK BAG

Valium for your own personal use

• • • • • • • • • • •

Worry beads

• • • • • • • • • • •

The board game *Operation*, which you use to practise your surgical technique

• • • • • • • • • • •

A large box of sweets ready to decant into pill bottles to fool gullible hypochondriacs

THINGS TO KEEP TELLING YOURSELF

One day I will be able to retire –
assuming I survive that long

• • • • • • • • • • •

I am doing an important job much valued by
the community – rather like a pub landlord

• • • • • • • • • • •

Even if all my patients diagnosed themselves
using the internet they would still have
to come to me for a second opinion

I WILL BE ABLE TO KEEP MY JOB FOR LIFE DESPITE THE FACT THAT ONE HUNDRED PER CENT OF MY PATIENTS WILL ULTIMATELY FAIL TO SURVIVE

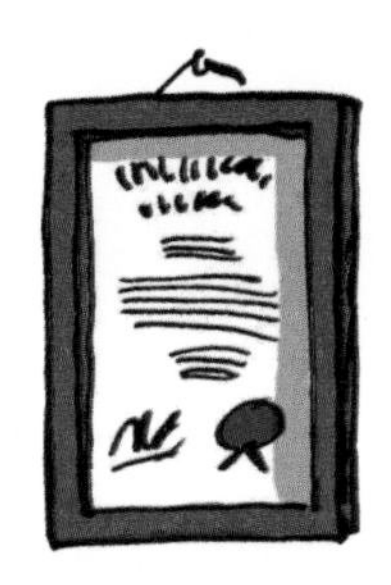